HOW I LOST 50 POUNDS WITHOUT EXERCISE! MY PERSONAL JOURNEY TO A HEALTHY WAY OF LIVING

ANNETT HILL

Disclaimer Notice and Terms of Use:

The information in this book is the opinion of the author and is base on the author's personal experiences and observations. The author does not assume any liability whatsoever for the use of, or the inability to use any or all information contained in this book, and accepts no responsibility for any loss or damages of any kind that may be incurred by the reader as a result of actions arising from the use of information found within this book. Use the information at your own risk. No promises of cures, capabilities, weight loss results or otherwise are given by the author herein.

Table of Contents

ACKNOWLEDGMENTS

Thanks to Jesus my Lord and Savior, who gave me the strength and endurance to go through such experience of losing the weight. There were times when I felt like quitting; it was not an easy road, but he kept me going. Thank you, Jesus! You are an awesome God.

I would also like to thank my husband and son who encouraged me when I was on my weight loss journey. They did not know it at the time, but they were supportive in one way or another. When I ate junk, my husband would lovingly encourage me not to; at the time, I did not appreciate his efforts, but I knew it was for my good. He loves me and wants what is best for me. I can honestly say that my husband never made me feel insecure in our relationship in any way. He loves me through thick and thin. For this, I am very much grateful.

I want to acknowledge my grandparents for loving me unconditionally; they never made me feel unloved in any way. May their souls rest in peace. To my family, thanks for cheering me on. I love you guys!

INTRODUCTION

Are you struggling with obesity? Have you tried to lose weight and cannot seem to make it happen? First, it is essential to know that you are not alone. Losing weight is a challenge. The good news is that there are numerous resources to help you manage weight loss and obesity. If you are someone like me who do not like to exercise, do not worry, you do not need it to accomplish weight loss. The best part, you will not have to deprive yourself to lose weight. There are healthy alternatives to unhealthy processed foods that you are accustom to eating. Losing weight has changed my life so much so, that I am compelled to write this book to help you. Keep reading to find out how you can lose the weight and change your life too. I am so happy to share my story of how I lost 50 pounds in 7 months without any form of exercise whatsoever. Yes, I did it! My goal in sharing my weight loss success is to help you if you are struggling to lose weight. I know the struggle, I have been there, and I know it can be very frustrating. I will tell you how I overcame that battle and what I did to lose the weight.

First, I must tell you about myself and how I became obese. The truth is, I never saw myself as obese; I thought I was a little overweight. Whatever I am going to share with you is base on my experience and results, I achieved these results because of what I did. I am neither a doctor nor a dietician; hence, I am not qualified to give medical advice. I am only sharing what I did and how you can implement what I share in your life too. Before you try any of these tips, please do your research first.

My name is Annett Hill. I was born and raised by my loving grandparents on the beautiful island of Jamaica. Sadly, they are now passed away, may their souls rest in peace. Life in Jamaica is terrific; we have many traditions, which foods are of significance. Traditional Sunday dinner is a must. One of the many Jamaican culinary traditions is to have Sunday dinner cooked every week in Jamaican households. The meal of rice and peas, meat and vegetables is a classic dinner that you will often find served on Sundays. We cook lots of starchy foods, dumplings, rice, yams and many bread products. We also made lots of sweet drinks and sweet pastries, such as cake, bun, and candies.

Growing up, I was on the chubby side, and so were most kids who were fat while growing up. The primary reason had to do with us eating lots of cookies, cake, ice cream, candies and other sugary foods. Do not get me wrong; we had plenty of fruits and vegetables also. We cultivated our vegetables and fruits, so we had plenty, and I ate plenty too. You see, in Jamaica when you are chubby, it is seen as being healthy, and it does not matter how big you are, you are thought to be healthy and enjoying life. On the other hand, if you are too skinny, you are considered malnourished and encouraged to eat more, during dinners your plate would be piled up with food all in an attempt to make you add more weight and look better off. Not to look malnourished, we would eat to maintain a "healthy" weight. Besides, we were taught not to waste food so if we get a plate of food we had to finish it. Even if we were full, our parents would say, "We work hard to provide food so don't waste it." You might ask why we did not leave some foods to eat later. Well, we were not allowed. They would say, "Eat up the food, do not leave any."

On December 26, 1988, I migrated to the United States of America; this was when everything changed with my eating habits. I remember the first time I tasted a snicker bar. Oh my! I loved it so much that from then on, I ate as many I could. I think I ate at least three bars every day, and yet I still craved for more. I ate plenty of peanut butter and crackers every day too, as well as other newly introduced junk food. In Jamaica, I did not have easy access to these things, and the opportunity I had; I made more than enough use of it, filling myself up with all sorts of junk. Soon enough, the junk food started creeping up on me, and I began to gain weight a lot. I then began different fad diets to lose weight. I took diet pills, which never worked, for me; they only made me sick in the stomach.

In 1990, I got pregnant with my only child and to my amazement; I started losing weight, which was unusual because most women gain weight when they are pregnant. My obstetrician would run tests to see why I was not gaining weight and was a little concerned that my baby would have a low birth weight. In 1991, I gave birth to a healthy 7lbs 3ozs baby boy; he did not have a low birth weight. In a twist of turns, I started gaining weight after my son was born. I joined the gym and began to cut back on the calories that I was consuming. I did lose some weight, but after a few months, I stopped cutting calories and also stopped going to the gym because I started to work as a live-in Home Health Aide. The weight started creeping back on, and I got to 200 pounds. I maintained this weight for years. In 1996, I came across Dr. Atkins Diet Revolution Book; I bought it and started to follow his diet, which is a Low Carbohydrate, and the Ketogenic Diet. I loved it because it worked. I lost about 20 pounds, and I felt great, but the only drawback was after I stopped eating the Low Carbohydrate meals, I gained back all the weight and even more. I also struggled with emotional eating, whenever I was stressed or sad, I turned to food, especially sweet pastries such as cake, cookies chocolate and hard candies.

It was in 2014; I started to think seriously about my health and my weight issue after my doctor told me my A1C level was 5.9. The A1C test is a blood test that provides information about your average levels of blood glucose, also called blood sugar, over the past three months. The A1C test can be used to diagnose type 2 diabetes and prediabetes. The A1C test is the primary test used for diabetes management.

An A1C level below 5.7 percent is considered normal. An A1C between 5.7 and 6.4 percent signals prediabetes. Type 2 diabetes diagnosed when the A1C is over 6.5 percent. She suggested that I cut out refined carbohydrates and sugar which I love. It was hard to do, but I did this for a little while, but not for long, remember I said earlier that I am an emotional eater. Yes, I would eat anything when I was stressed out. I know this type of behavior is not healthy and I have to get it under control. I still today struggle with it, but I am learning how to control the urge to eat when I am stress. Many of us eat because we are unhappy. If you are struggling with the emotions of obesity or past traumas, consider getting help. Once you can come to terms with your feelings, you can begin to control your eating habits. You can live a happy, healthy and fulfilling life.

It was April of 2016 that I got serious about losing weight. It all started when my co-workers decided to start a weight loss challenge, and the winner would get a monetary prize. I was reluctant to join them, but one of my coworkers encouraged me. "It would be fun," she told me. I said yes, and at that moment, I knew there was no turning back, the game was on. I have to admit the money was a good motivation also. There were three prizes for the first, second, and third positions. I knew I wanted the first prize, so if I was going to win; I had to take losing weight seriously. I am a big competitor; I knew I had to win; I was going to do everything within my power, and push my limits to win. I began to research; I already knew about Ketogenic and Low Carbohydrates Diet and that they worked, but I needed to know more than I did to get to my goal. I knew that after I lost weight, I would need to maintain it. I think this is the biggest hurdle. My problem was never to lose weight; it was maintenance. I was always on Google, Pinterest and YouTube researching; these platforms became my best friends.

The weight loss challenge started April 19, 2016, and ran through July 12, 2016. My goal was to lose 50 pounds overall. I had never lost that much weight before, but I was willing to try. I wanted to do it healthily by losing 2 pounds per week, which would be 24 pounds at the end of the challenge. My goal also depended on the other competitors' progress; if they were losing more than that, then I would have to aim for more. I started with the Ketogenic Diet because I knew it works. I went cold turkey by drastically cutting out all refined carbohydrates and sugar, this was very hard, but I had to so I could lose the weight. For breakfast, I would eat bacon and eggs; sometimes I would have cheese with it. Lunch would be some form of meat kind with vegetables. I replaced the rice and dumplings with vegetables. Dinner would pretty much be the same type of foods I ate for lunch. I kept it simple until later on, I got creative with meals. I did not want to be bored with foods by eating the same thing repeatedly. I had to cook for my husband and son, and this was very hard. We Jamaicans love the whole heap of starchy foods, like the dumplings, yams, and rice.

We had to weigh in every Tuesday; the first weigh-in was to determine our weight. I started with the weight of 206 pounds. The first week of the challenge I lost 5 pounds, I was shocked at losing that much in one week, I knew it was mostly water weight anyway. Losing that much weight gave me the drive to continue. The second week I lost 3 pounds, the third week I lost 2 pounds, then in subsequent weeks, I lost about 1.5 pounds per week. As long as I was losing weight every week, I was ok with it. I was the only one that had weight loss every weigh in. Some people would gain a few pounds here and there. It motivated me even more. At a point, it was no longer about winning anymore, sure, I wanted to win, but seeing how many pounds I was losing made me feel encouraged, it made me want to reach my setout goals notwithstanding if I was going to win or not. It was now a month after I started the weight loss and was down 11.5 pounds.

I was beginning to feel much better with my body; I was now able to fit into some smaller clothes, which I still had over the years in my closet that I had bought when I was on a roller-coaster diet. I had hopes of fitting into the smaller clothes one day, so I kept them. I had three different dress sizes in my closet. Size 16, size 14 and size 12. I was wearing the size 16 dress when I started the weight loss journey. I was now able to fit into size 14 clothes. I was on cloud nine, and this led me to lose even some more weight. Now I did not feel tired and sluggish like I had felt before, and this was a bonus. During my research, I came across Intermittent Fasting by Dr. Fung, which I incorporated in my journey; this helped a lot. I did the Intermittent Fast every day; I did the 16:8 protocol, with this, I fasted for 16 hours and ate within the 8-hour window. I would stop eating at 8 pm and did not eat until the next day at noon. I will discuss later this fasting protocol. I still was researching because I needed to learn everything I could to know how to maintain weight loss. I also came across Wheat Belly Diet by Dr. Davis. I will explain in details later about this diet too.

July 12, 2016, was the end of the weight loss challenge at my job. It was the final weigh in. I lost 23 pounds, and I was the first prize winner. The second prize winner lost 11 pounds and the third prize winner lost 8 pounds, both of them not even measuring up with how many pounds I had lost. I fitted my size 12 clothes; I was thrilled and glad that I had gotten myself involved in the challenge; I had never thought I could push myself that hard before. It just shows that whatever you put your mind to; you will succeed. I had not reached the 50lbs goal that I wanted to lose, but I was not going to give up. I bought a scale and continued with my weight-loss journey with the mindset that I had 27 pounds to go. I did not set a goal of how many pounds I wanted to lose each week at that time, all I knew was that I needed to drop an extra 27 pounds to make it 50. Every Saturday I would weigh myself to make sure that I was achieving weight loss. I continued the weight loss journey with the different types of diets I found. The Wheat Belly Diet, Ketogenic Diet, and Intermittent Fasting. As mentioned earlier, I will discuss later in detail about each of these methods so you can use also.

I lost the additional 27 pounds in 4 months, which ended November 21, 2016. I lost an average of 1.5 lbs per week, and although in the beginning I had said I wanted to lose 2 pounds per week, it did not happen that way. The greatest thing is that I was losing weight every week, when you decided to lose weight do not restrict yourself to a certain amount per week, you may lose 1 pound some weeks, you may lose 3 pounds other weeks, and another week you may lose only 0.5 pounds. You see, when you put a restriction on how much weight you want to lose, you may be disappointed if you do not lose that amount each week; this can be stressful and might cause you to give up. Even though I did not do any form of exercise, this does not mean I am against it. I am only telling you how I lost weight without workouts; if you want to implement activity go right ahead. I did not start doing exercises until after I lost the weight. The fact remains, we do not need it to lose weight, but it is good for our overall health. I do not like to workout, and I have to admit that my favorite exercise is dancing, but now and then, I do a little weight lifting, squats, and planks. I had lost 50 lbs! I made it! Soon came the best part, the shopping spree.

Going shopping is the best part of losing weight; it was definitely worth all the sacrifices. I did not have much money, and although I was limited in my choices, it was fun. I remember the first day I walked into Sears Department Store to try on clothes. I had waited to lose the 50 pounds before I started shopping, so I was wearing the size 12 clothes; I still had in my closet even though they were loose on me. I was looking at getting size 8-10 clothes or medium because I figured that would be the size that would fit me. They, however, seemed small to me; the last time I had worn medium size clothes had been in high school, and I greatly doubted they would fit me. I took four dresses in the fitting room with doubts that I would fit into them, but to my surprise, the dresses fit perfectly. I was looking so sexy and fabulous in front of the mirrors that I did not want to take the clothes off. I did not have to suck in my stomach to make it look flat; this was one of the things I used to do to make my tummy looked flat, including wearing tummy cinchers. Although I was excited about my new clothes, I was even more excited to get back home, so I bought the dresses and went home. I tried them on for my husband and asked him to take a photograph; this was the first picture I took since I started the weight loss journey. When I saw the picture, I was so amazed; I could not believe what I saw. I put it next to a photo I had taken a few months before I started the weight loss journey. It looked like I had lost half of my body size. I was in tears and could not believe that I had done it. I had accomplished what I had set out to do splendidly.

Now I want to help you, the fact that you are reading this book means you or someone you may know and love is struggling with weight issues; I want to be a voice and inspiration. My mission is to help you and everyone else who is struggling with obesity. I have been there, I have tried many diets, and while some worked, some did not. I believe I know now what works for losing weight. I will suggest before starting any diet program to consult your doctor first. Also, everyone will have different results; we are all different and no matter what the results are, do not give up. You are beautiful no matter what size you are; you deserve to be the best by being healthy. I know we as humans like instant gratification, we love a quick fix. I encourage you to do it slowly, try losing up to 2 pounds per week. Slow and steady is the best way. I see many diets that claim to lose 10 pounds in one week, I am not saying it is impossible, but I believe it is too much in such a short time. It is mostly water anyway; you do not lose fat. Your goal should be to lose fat. Some people want to take some pills and wish the weight gone. I am sure we did not gain all the weight overnight, so why do we expect to lose it overnight? We have to be realistic in our approach to weight loss. Weight loss overnight is only a pipe dream. I tried it; it does not work.

There are people that I know for years, who saw how much weight I have lost don't believe I lost all this weight by only changing the way I eat. When I explained what I did, that I cut out all refined carbohydrates and sugar they looked at me as if I was crazy. "That's it? Can't be!" They went ahead to ask me what pill I took or what surgery I did. We do not know that we are what we eat. I struggled with weight issues most of my adult life, and I know it is frustrating. At times, I did not like to look in the mirror. I refrained from going out because I did not like how I looked in my clothes. I never shared these feelings with anyone, my family and friends thought I did not want to go out, or at least I led them to believe so. It was when I lost weight I confessed to my husband the truth why I never wanted to go out. I am so passionate about helping you and others gain knowledge on how you can lose weight. It is not as hard as it seems, I can honestly say this now.

Whenever I see someone who is obese, all I want to do now is to help. I do wish I could stop those people I see on the street or the subway, to give some advice. I know I cannot. I would not want anyone to tell me I am fat. I wish I could do something to help, which is why I am writing this book. I know there are many weight loss books on the market, but I do hope as you read this book you will see that there is real hope of losing weight. I do believe that the way to lose fat is cutting refined carbohydrates and sugar. To prove that I want to help, I am sharing with you my email. If you wish to talk or have any questions, do not hesitate, send me an email. howilost50pounds@gmail.com

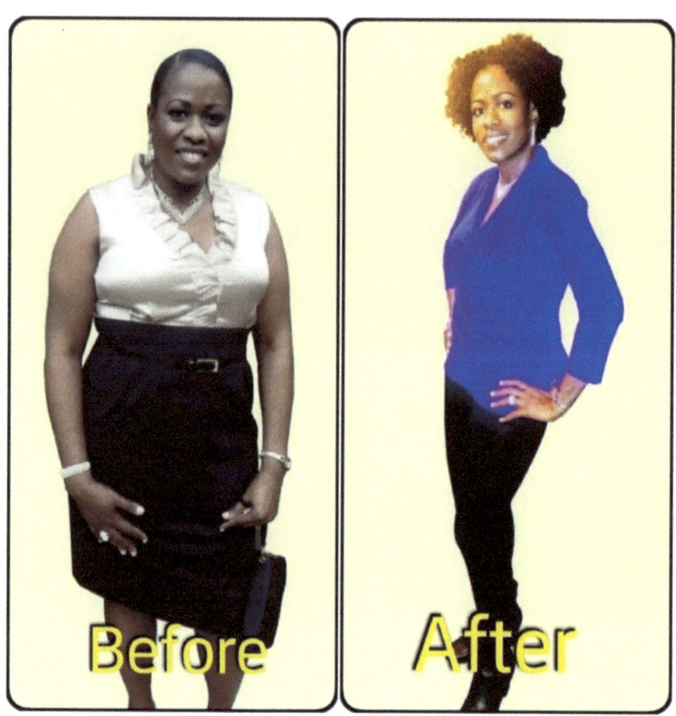

OBESITY GETTING WORSE

Obesity affects almost 30% of the adult population. It also affects about 25% of our youth. It is causing problems everywhere, from the cost of health care to legislation; it affects every one of us. You are probably already aware that obesity has reached epidemic proportions. However, you may not be familiar with these surprising obesity statistics. According to data collected by the CDC where you live has a direct effect on your obesity risk.

People who live in the southern United States have the highest risk for obesity. More than 30% of the population in the south is obese. Second, only to the Midwest, this has between 25% and 29% obesity rate. Colorado has the lowest incidence of obesity in the United States with fifteen to nineteen % of the population being obese and while it seems like the US has cornered the market on obesity that is not necessarily true. Mexico, the United Kingdom, Greece, Slovakia, New Zealand and Australia all have a high obesity rate.

The countries with the lowest obesity percentage rate are South Korea and Japan both tie for the lowest with just 3.2% of the population. Obesity is a problem around the globe. It does not matter what your race or religion is; the numbers continue to grow. As it grows, so do the financial and health costs. In fact, according to a study conducted by the CDC, the direct and indirect cost of obesity costs $147 billion annually.

The study also found that obese patients spend an average of $1,429 more for their medical care than people within a healthy weight range do. There is good news in all of this. Obesity has gained attention over the past few years. Therefore, a solution will be imminent. People struggling with obesity have more support and solutions than ever before. If you are struggling with obesity, there is hope. There is help

What is Obesity?

Are You Obese or Overweight? Learn The Difference. With obesity at historic highs, one might assume that most people are obese. It is true that one in three people are obese. However, there is a vast difference between obese and overweight. Let us explore the basics. There are a few ways to determine obesity. Some physicians look strictly at the weight. Others look at the percentage of body fat a person has. For example, if you have more than 30% body fat, then you are considered obese.

Thirty percent of your body is fat, not muscle, bone, blood or other tissue. However, the most commonly used form to define obesity is a BMI calculation. It is a simple equation that essentially compares weight to height. If you have a BMI or Body Mass Index of 30 or more, then you are considered obese. IF you have a BMI of 40 or more, then you are considered morbidly obese. Yet, if you have a BMI of 25-29, then you are considered overweight. My BMI was 34, so I was deemed obese.

How to Calculate Your BMI

1. Multiply your height in inches times your height in inches.
2. Divide your weight by the number you arrived at in Step 1.
3. Multiply the number you came up with in Step 2 by 705.
4. The result is your BMI.

You might be surprised to know that more than 30% of the country is overweight. This coupled with the 30% obesity rate means that more than sixty percent of the population is overweight or obese. Two out of every three people are carrying more weight than is healthy for their body. According to the World Health Organization, one billion people are overweight or obese globally. This number has doubled in the past few decades.

Cause of Obesity

Our lives are changing. Access to food is quick and easy now, and it is cheap. Stop by any fast food restaurant, and you can fill your belly for just a few dollars. Unfortunately, those few dollars add a lot of sugar, sodium, and fat to your body. One fast food stop can provide all of the calories and sugar you need for the entire day. However, most people do not eat just once a day. That means they are consuming more calories than they are burning. It only takes an extra hundred calories a day to cause you to gain a pound a month. Also, as the numbers are showing, most people are consuming more than an extra hundred calories a day. Chances are you know someone struggling with obesity. Approximately one in three people are obese, and the numbers are rising. You may even be struggling with it yourself.

These intakes of high-calorie foods and beverages with an inactive lifestyle and you have a recipe for weight gain. True, diet and fitness levels are not the only causes of obesity. However, they are the primary causes. Scientists agree that some people can be genetically predisposed to obesity. Diet and exercise still control weight. Medications, mental and physical health issues also contribute to obesity. Add it all up; it is easy to see why more than half of the country and much of the world is overweight.

There is a solution regardless of the factors causing obesity. There are two things you can do to improve your health. Get active, and change your eating habits. It is not easy. You will need to make lifestyle changes. However, your health is at risk if you are overweight or obese. In fact, your life is at risk. Take control of your life today. Start taking steps to get healthy.

How to Prevent Obesity

Studies have shown that there are "weight regulating" genes that seem to contribute to obesity. These genes regulate hormone release, control food intake or hunger, and control metabolism. Leptin, one of the hormones that control appetite, is regulated by a gene. Thus, it is easy to see that a person can inherit a good leptin regulating system or an ineffective leptin regulating system. If you suspect genetics are contributing to your obesity, look at your family history. Are your parents obese? What about your siblings? Grandparents? Does your family suffer from heart disease, high blood pressure, strokes or high cholesterol? If they do, chances are you may have a genetic predisposition to obesity. Genes are not The Predominating Factor in Obesity.

While genetics may play a role in your predisposition to obesity, Diet and lifestyle are still the primary contributors. If you eat lots of refined carbohydrates and sugar, you are going to gain weight. Therefore, if you have a leptin imbalance and are always feeling hungry, you have to look at other lifestyle and eating habits to support a healthy weight. For example, eating foods that promote healthy leptin levels, and eating foods that are high in fiber also help. For example, eating an apple for a snack instead of potato chips. Exercise also plays a vital role in balancing hormones and metabolism.

The hard truth is that lifestyle choices cause most obesity. For most people, lifestyle choices are learned. Parents help set the foundation for a child to live a healthy life and to make healthy decisions. Obese children often have obese parents, because of poor lifestyle choices. A lifetime of poor habits can add up. The good news is that you can change poor habits. Lifestyle choices can be modified to support good health and weight loss.

Five Effects of Obesity

Most people know that obesity is the leading cause of type 2 diabetes. They should also know that it causes many types of cancer. It causes heart disease, stroke, high blood pressure, and death. Overall, obesity causes many health problems. Obesity is said to be one of the highest causes of death in the United States. Obesity is reversible. You do not have to live with these health complications hanging over your head. Consult your physician and get on a program today to start living a healthier life. However, you might be surprised to know that obesity causes some other day-to-day effects. Here are some of them.

1. Depression

Depression and obesity have a very tight connection. It has theorized that depression causes obesity. However, it is a known fact that obesity causes depression in many individuals. The reason is complicated. Often, people lose their self-esteem and confidence when they are obese. Especially in the case of teenagers and young children who may be facing teasing at school. However, obesity also contributes to the inability of a person to get good sleep. It can cause many sleep disorders. Sleep apnea, for example, is often caused by obesity.

When a person is not able to get quality sleep, their brain chemistry can change. Poor sleep often leads to depression. Additionally, obesity is often contributed to by inactivity. Activity and exercise release feel-good hormones. These hormones will not release in inactive people. The result can be a depression or a chronic bad mood.

2. Poor Sleep and Sleep Disorders

Obesity also causes some sleep disorders. Sleep is crucial for healthy physical and mental functioning. Inadequate sleep causes irritability and depression. It causes poor functioning. It also creates a weakened immune system. Furthermore, insufficient sleep causes a person to gain weight. The good news is that merely getting seven hours of sleep each night can make a world of difference.

3. Skin Problems.

Obesity affects metabolism. It also affects hormone levels and organ functioning. Specifically, it can cause reduced liver function or fatty liver disease. When your liver is not functioning well, your skin can pay the price. Changes in hormones may cause Acanthosis Nigricans, which are dark velvety areas of the neck and body folds, while stretching of the skin may result in stretch marks. Increased strain on the leg veins may cause fluid retention, leg swelling, rupture of superficial capillaries, and varicose veins. You can break out with acne. You can even suffer skin infections due to a weakened immune system.

4. Hair and Nails.

An obese body is struggling to function optimally. Because of that, several functions are ignored to take care of the primary functions of your heart and lungs. Quite quickly, you may notice that your hair changes. It may start to fall out. It may change in texture and become coarse and brittle. Your nails may also grow brittle and yellow because of the weakened immune system and poor liver function.

5. Decreased Sexual Interest and Function.

Libido and sexual function can drastically decrease in obese people. In fact, many obese people find it extremely difficult to get pregnant; because the hormone levels are imbalanced. Fat cells produce hormones. They also inhibit balanced hormone production. Your desire to have sex will decrease. If you are trying to have children, you may also struggle with fertility problems. Finally, many obese women suffer from gynecological issues like ovarian cysts and endometriosis. If you are struggling with obesity, there is help. You can regain your health and vitality.

Treatments for Obesity

The treatments for obesity are varied. They depend on the person, the cause of the obesity and the seriousness of the person's health. Treatment ranges from lifestyle changes diet and exercise to surgery. If you are obese, it is important to lose weight. Obesity brings with it a whole host of health risks. Many of these risks are life-threatening. To treat and manage obesity meet with your doctor to create a treatment plan. Obesity is not a life sentence. You can lose weight and regain your health and vitality. The first step is understanding what obesity is. The second step is getting a diagnosis. Finally, create a treatment plan and begin the path to your healthier future.

Dietary Changes

In any situation, your physician will make specific dietary changes. Even if you undergo surgery or take medication, you will need to change your diet. What you eat has a direct impact on your weight. How much you eat does as well. Common changes include severely reducing sugary baked goods and processed foods. You will replace them with protein, lots of fiber, fruits, vegetables and good fats. The idea is to make lifestyle changes that are sustainable. Dieting is a short-term solution.

Behavior Change

You will likely be asked to change some habits. For example, your physician may ask you to get more sleep. They may ask you to cut back on alcohol or kick other habits.

Prescription Weight-Loss Medications

In some instances, your doctor may prescribe a medication to help you lose weight. Diet and exercise will still be part of the program. Medication is not for everyone. There are some side effects and risks.

Weight-Loss Surgery

Surgery is a treatment solution if you are facing immediate health risks due to obesity, the operation may be your solution. It requires a high degree of commitment. After you have had weight loss surgery, there is no going back. You will experience some side effects. You will also have to make many lifestyle changes. It does, however, provide a viable solution for those who are severely obese. If you are struggling with obesity, consult with your physician. Together you can create a plan to get healthy. Sad, isn't it? I was one of such figures for obesity, but I have been able to make it out of the alarming statistics. Now let me tell you about the three methods I incorporated into my weight loss journey so you can start today

THIS IS THE DAY, WHICH THE LORD HATH MADE; LET US REJOICE AND BE GLAD IN IT. PSALM 118:24

KETOGENIC DIET

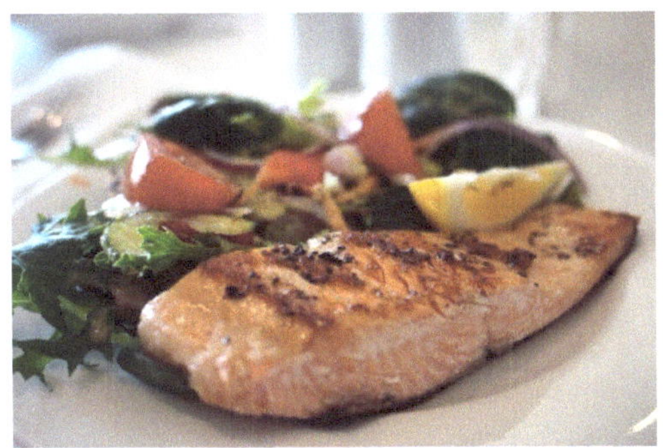

Of all the diets, the Ketogenic Diet is my favorite. I love Ketogenic Diet because I can eat real foods, including meats, eggs, nuts, seeds and good fats. I was never hungry on this diet. Preparing a meal for this diet was easy. All I had to do was to eliminate refined carbohydrates and sugar. I did not eat any products made with white flour. I will share some of my favorite ketogenic recipes at the end of this book in the recipes section. For more in-depth knowledge of the Ketogenic Diet, check this website out.

https://draxe.com/hub/keto-diet/

What is the Ketogenic Diet?

The fundamental principle of the Ketogenic Diet is that a state of ketosis will help you burn your fat stores as energy. Many people, even those who are on a Low Carbohydrate Diet, do not quite understand ketosis and why it works. Most diets are calorie-reduction diets. They help you lose weight, but some of the weight is from fat, and some of it is from lean muscle tissue. While you may look smaller on the scale, your metabolism is slowing down. The more muscle you lose, the slower your metabolism will be. Losing weight will be more difficult and gaining weight back even simpler. The Ketogenic Diet is carbohydrate restrictive. It creates a state of ketosis in your body that burns only fat, and not muscle. The primary source of your energy for your body will be fat in the form of ketones. Your liver will convert fat into ketones, and it cannot convert back. It will excrete naturally.

What is Ketones?

Ketones are a normal and efficient source of fuel for the human body. The liver creates it from the fatty acids that result from the breakdown of body fat. These only appear when there is an absence of glucose and sugar. In the Ketogenic Diet, you reduce the amount of glucose and sugar that is in the bloodstream. As a result, your body produces ketones for fuel. When your body is creating ketones, it is called ketosis. There is a common misconception that following a Ketogenic Diet is dangerous. The truth is that being in ketosis is a completely natural state. The human body creates ketones to use as fuel in the absence of glucose. Reaching a state of ketosis is vital to success on the Ketogenic Diet and it as simple as eliminating carbohydrates and sugar from the diet

How to Get Into Ketosis

Cut down on consuming glucose from carbohydrate foods, grains, starchy vegetables, fruit, etc. Doing so forces your body to find an alternative fuel source: fat (think avocados, coconut oil, and salmon). Meanwhile, in the absence of glucose, the body also starts to burn fat and produces ketones instead. Once ketone levels in the blood rise to a certain point, you enter into a state of ketosis. This state of high ketone levels results in quick and consistent weight loss until you reach a healthy, stable body weight

You may be wondering how many carb foods you may eat and still be in ketosis. The classic Ketogenic Diet made for all those with epilepsy consisted to getting about 75 percent of calories in sources of fat (such as oils or fattier cuts of meat), 5 percent by carbs and 20 percent from protein. For most people, a less strict Ketogenic Diet can help boost weight loss in a safe and often very fast manner.

To transition and remain in ketosis, the recommended amount of total net grams of carbs you should start with is about 30–50 net grams. Beginning with this approach is more moderate and flexible but can be less overwhelming. Once you are more accustomed to this way of eating, you can choose to lower carbs even more if you would like, down to about 20 grams of net carbs daily. The 20 gram is the standard, "strict" amount that many Keto dieters aim to adhere to for best results, but remember that everyone is a bit different.

How Do You Benefit On The Ketogenic Diet?

Weight Loss: Go from sugar burner to fat burner. Release less insulin so less fat storage. Significantly reduces appetite

Reduce Risk for Type 2 Diabetes: Prevent excessive insulin release. Create a normal blood sugar level

Fight Heart Disease: Lower (LDL) Cholesterol. Lower triglyceride

Cancer: The diet is currently being used to treat several types of cancer and slow tumor growth.

Alzheimer's Disease: The diet may reduce symptoms of Alzheimer's and slow down the disease's progression.

Epilepsy: Research has shown that the Ketogenic Diet can cause massive reductions in seizures in epileptic children.

Parkinson's Disease: One study found that the diet helped improve symptoms of Parkinson's disease.

Polycystic ovary syndrome: The Ketogenic Diet can help reduce insulin levels, which may play a key role in polycystic ovary syndrome.

Acne: Lower insulin levels and eating less sugar or processed foods may help improve acne.

What Can You Eat On The Ketogenic Diet?

Meat- (such as beef, pork, veal, lamb) just about any cut or preparation, though check the carbohydrates content of processed meat products like sausages and ensure you don't buy anything cured with sugar or honey.

Poultry- (chicken, turkey, quail, duck, etc.). It is preferable to leave the skin on poultry to increase the fat content. Poultry must not be breaded or battered, but can otherwise be prepared any way you like, roasted, stir-fried, deep fried, baked, grilled or barbecued.

Fish and Shellfish- They should be fresh, things like imitation crabmeat often contain added carbohydrates – and if you buy, canned fish make sure it has not been preserved with added sugar. Again, it must not be breaded or battered.

Eggs- You will probably find that eggs become a staple when you are on a Ketogenic Diet.

Cheese- Most types of cheese are suitable for a Ketogenic Diet, though they do contain some carbohydrates, so make sure you include these in your daily carbohydrates count to ensure you stay below your limit.

Vegetables- Vegetables will be the source of most of the carbohydrates you eat, but you still need to choose the lowest carbohydrates vegetables with the best nutritional value.

Green leafy vegetables are the best, such as spinach, all kinds of lettuce and cabbage, watercress, brussels sprouts, and kale. You can also eat broccoli and cauliflower, celery, cucumber, asparagus, bean sprouts, radishes and more, but must strictly limit your intake of sugary vegetables like peppers, onions, and tomatoes, and avoid starchy vegetables like potatoes.

Nuts- Almond, walnuts, macadamia, and pecans can eat in moderation as a snack.

Oils- Coconut oil, olive oil, and butter can use in cooking.

Fresh herbs and dry spices- can use for flavor.

Mayonnaise and oil-based salad dressings- are usually ok, but check the carbohydrates content on the bottle.

Artificial Sweetener- such as stevia and monk fruit sweetener can use in place of sugar.

Foods to Limit on the Ketogenic Diet:

Some select foods that may be lower carb but can still push you over the 20–30 net carbs per day threshold, so these are the foods that you need to limit when going on a Keto Diet

- Full-fat dairy (opt for unsweetened almond milk or coconut milk instead)
- Medium-starchy veggies like sweet peas, carrots, beets and any potatoes
- Legumes and beans
- Nuts and seeds

Foods to Avoid On the Keto Diet

You must avoid these foods when compiling your meal plans:

- Any types of sugar, including natural sugars like raw honey or maple syrup (sorry!)
- Any grains, including oats, rice, quinoa, pasta and corn
- All processed foods, including crackers, candy, cookies, ice cream, snack bars and canned soup
- Sweetened and caloric beverages, including alcohol and milk
- Products label Low fat, Low calorie

HE WHO DOES NOT LOVE DOES NOT KNOW GOD, FOR GOD IS LOVE. IN THIS, THE LOVE OF GOD WAS MANIFESTED TOWARD US, THAT GOD HAS SENT HIS ONLY BEGOTTEN SON INTO THE WORLD, THAT WE MIGHT LIVE THROUGH HIM. IN THIS IS LOVE, NOT THAT WE LOVED GOD, BUT THAT HE LOVED US AND SENT HIS SON TO BE THE PROPITIATION FOR OUR SINS." 1 JOHN 4:8-10

WHEAT BELLY DIET

The second diet is the Wheat Belly Diet. I struggled at first because cutting out wheat was the biggest hurdle with this diet. Going wheat free meant no more bagel, bread pancake, and cookies, or so I thought. Then I realized after much more research I could still eat all these things, but I have to use wheat-free flours. I can no longer use any types of wheat flours. I found out about Coconut Flour, Almond Flour, and Flaxseed Meal. I never knew these types of flours existed. You will still need to eat in moderation. These flours still have carbohydrates. I will share some wheat free recipes for you to try at the end of the book. These recipes will help you to maintain this lifestyle. For more in-depth knowledge of the Wheat Belly Diet, check this website out.
http://www.wheatbellyblog.com/

What is Wheat Belly Diet?

The Wheat Belly Diet is a dietary plan created by cardiologist William Davis, M.D., which excludes all sources of wheat, which means the majority of high-calorie, packaged foods are off-limits. Haven't people been eating wheat for thousands of years, you might be wondering? Moreover, aren't "whole wheat" products supposed to be healthy? Dr. Davis wrote in his book "Wheat Belly" that what most people think of as wheat or whole wheat is not wheat at all, but more like a type of transformed grain product that's the result of genetic research conducted during the latter half of the 20th century. He argued that eating lots of modern-day wheat is one of the leading causes of health problems. Excluding wheat from your diet also means that most (or even all) of the gluten in your diet is removed, which according to some researches can be beneficial for things like improving digestive health and in some cases reducing inflammation levels and boosting immunity. Gluten is a type of protein found in grains, including all varieties of wheat (like kamut or wheat berries), plus barley and rye. It makes up about 80 percent of the amino acids (the building blocks of proteins) found in these grains and is believed to contribute to a variety of symptoms of gluten intolerance or food allergies that might affect millions of people.

Why Go Wheat Free?

Let us talk about what might happen when you stop eating wheat. There is a very good chance that you have been living with symptoms that you thought were just a part of life. Some of these symptoms are bloating, migraines, and allergies. When you stop eating wheat, these symptoms are going to disappear, and you are going to experience an entirely new level of life and vitality. I know this is true because it happened to me. How do you eat a sandwich without wheat? You do not. You can make wheat free bread with wheat-free flours, such as Coconut, Almond and Flaxseed Meal.

Benefits of Wheat Free

Better Skin – For many people, acne is an immune response or a side effect of a compromised immune system. If your body has to choose between protecting your internal organs or letting you get a few pimples, guess what? You are getting the pimples. Going wheat free reduces the immune strain on your body. If you have eczema or psoriasis, you will likely see an improvement too.

Weight Loss – People who cut wheat out of their diet lose weight. They lose it for a variety of reasons. One, your diet is healthier because you are not eating so many starchy carbohydrates, which are empty calories. Two, these same carbohydrates also lead to insulin resistance, which causes your body to eat more and crave sugar, so you get calories and energy to your cells. You overeat in an attempt to supply your cells with energy. Three, you are eliminating a protein in wheat, gliadin, that has been shown to be an appetite stimulant. Finally, wheat and the corresponding immune response cause systemic inflammation. Your body essentially swells up. When your body no longer has to fight, the swelling goes down, and you look and feel thinner.

More Energy – You are going to be surprised how much energy you have when you cut wheat out of your diet. You will sleep more soundly. Your blood sugar levels will stay more even, and your body will not be spending all its time battling the effects of wheat. You will have the energy to spare. People who cut wheat out of their lives also enjoy:

- Fewer headaches
- Improved digestion
- Improved mood
- Fewer aches and pains
- Improved allergy symptoms

And much more. I know that when I stopped eating wheat my seasonal allergies practically disappeared and I stopped experiencing weekly migraines; I was also experiencing debilitating fatigue and gastrointestinal problems that no one should have to face. I sleep like a baby, and I wake up feeling energetic. That energy lasts all day. It has changed my life, and it will change yours too.

Steps to Eliminating Wheat from Your Diet

Did you know that your soy sauce probably contains wheat? Your lipstick might be too. Most of us are naive about how many foods contain wheat and gluten. Yes, I know lipstick is not food, but if you wear it, then you ingest it. It happens when you lick your lips or eat something that touches your lips. Probably not a big deal unless you are allergic to gluten. Let us get back to that soy sauce. Wheat is typically an ingredient in soy sauce. It is also in an abundance of other foods you probably would not expect to see it in including.

- Soups
- Cereals
- Crackers
- Salad Dressings
- Pasta
- Potato Chips
- French Fries
- Energy Bars
- Candy and Candy bars
- Tortilla Chips
- Brown Rice Syrup
- Meat substitutes like Veggie Burgers
- Pre-seasoned meats like Rotisserie Chickens and many Types of lunch meats.

Some of the foods on the list make sense, right? Pasta is made from flour, so it makes sense that it contains wheat. But what about things like French fries, tortilla chips, and meat? Why do they have wheat in them? It depends on the food but many foods contain wheat starch for thickening, or they contain things like malt. Malt is made from soaking grains in water and then drying them. Malted milkshakes, for example, have wheat in them. Therefore, the trick to avoiding wheat is to look on the label. Look for things like wheat, flour, starch, and malt. But what if you are avoiding gluten? Then the path gets a little trickier. And here is the thing, if you are going through the process to eliminate wheat, then it only makes sense to eliminate gluten too. Here is why. The vast majority of people who have problems with wheat do so because of the gluten. Yes, there are other reasons why people have problems with wheat. However, if you only eliminate wheat, you may not experience the benefits. Eliminate gluten, which is found in some additional foods and grains, and you will be sure to get rid of any aggravating proteins. At the grocery, you will find gluten in beer, vinegar, food coloring, condiments, and even some dairy products like cheesecake filling. Get used to reading labels. Look for signs on products that say "gluten-free." Whole Foods make Gluten Free easy.

If you eat many packaged and processed foods then eliminating wheat and gluten is going to be a tremendously rewarding lifestyle change. You can make the transition a whole lot easier on yourself by directly heading to the produce section of your market. Because here is the thing, other than grains, gluten does not naturally occur in other plants or animals. You can eat any meat, fruit, or vegetable without worrying about gluten.

BE STRONG AND OF GOOD COURAGE, FEAR NOT, NOR BE AFRAID FOR THE LORD THY GOD, HE IT IS THAT DOTH GO WITH THEE; HE WILL NOT FAIL THEE, NOR FORSAKE THEE. DEUTERONOMY 31:6

LAY UP FOR YOURSELVES TREASURES IN HEAVEN, WHERE NEITHER MOTH NOR RUST DOTH CORRUPT, AND WHERE THIEVES DO NOT BREAK THROUGH NOR STEAL: FOR WHERE YOUR TREASURE IS, THERE WILL YOUR HEART BE ALSO. MATTHEW 6:20-21

I WILL SAY OF THE LORD HE IS MY REFUGE AND MY FORTRESS: IN HIM WILL I TRUST. PSALM 91:2

INTERMITTENT FASTING

Intermittent Fasting is not a diet per say. On my weight loss journey, I used this fasting every day; I still do today, but not on a daily basis. Now, I fast for five days per week. I love Intermittent Fasting now, but when I first started, it was hard because I am accustomed to eating three meals a day especially breakfast, as I was forced to believe that breakfast is the most important meal of the day. It comes naturally now to fast, and I do not get hungry. I do the 16:8 fast, on this fast you do not eat for 16 hours, and then you have an 8 hours window eating time. I usually start my fasting at 8 pm to noon the next day. For more in-depth knowledge of the Intermittent Fasting, check this website out.
https://www.dietdoctor.com/intermittent-fasting

What is Intermittent Fasting?

It is a fact that Intermittent Fasting works. It has plenty of benefits besides weight loss. It reduces the risk of cancer, lowers blood pressure levels, reduces oxidative stress, and lowers bad cholesterol levels and so much more. No matter which type of Intermittent Fasting protocol you decide to go with, you can expect to enjoy some of the benefits of this fantastic method of eating. As for weight loss, deciding which style you go with is a very personal one.

You need to understand the fundamentals of Intermittent Fasting. The shorter the eating window, generally, the more fat you will burn. Fat loss occurs because your body is in a fasted state for a more extended period. If we start eating the minute we roll out of bed and do not stop until we go to sleep, we spend almost all our time in the fed state. Over time, we will gain weight because we have not allowed our body any time to burn food energy. Secondly, you will still need to be at a caloric deficit to see weight loss. Now, let us look at the common types of Intermittent Fasting.

3 Most Popular Methods of Intermittent Fasting

The 16/8 Method:

The 16/8 Method involves fasting every day for 14-16 hours and restricting your daily "eating window" to 8-10 hours. Within the eating window, you can fit in two, three or more meals. This method is also known as the Leangains protocol popularizes by fitness expert Martin Berkhan. Doing this method of fasting can be as simple as not eating anything after dinner, and skipping breakfast.

For example, if you finish your last meal at 8 pm and then do not eat until noon the next day, then you are technically fasting for 16 hours between meals. Women are recommended to only fast 14-15 hours because they seem to do better with slightly shorter fasts. For people who get hungry in the morning and like to eat breakfast, then this can be hard to get used to at first. However, many breakfast skippers instinctively eat this way. You can drink water, coffee without sugar, and other non-caloric beverages during the fast and this can help reduce hunger levels.

Eating mostly healthy foods during your eating window is essential. If you eat lots of junk food or excessive amounts of calories, weight loss will not occur. I find this to be the most "natural" way to do Intermittent Fasting. I eat this way myself and find it to be 100% effortless. I eat my last meal around 7-8 pm; I do not feel hungry until around 1 pm the next day, so I end up fasting for 17-18 hours.

Eat-Stop-Eat:

Eat-Stop-Eat involves 24-hour fast, either once or twice per week. Fitness expert Brad Pilon popularized this method and has been quite popular for a few years. By fasting from dinner one day, to dinner the next, this amounts to a 24-hour fast. For example, if you finish dinner on Sunday at 7 pm, and do not eat until dinner the next day at 7 pm, then you have just done a full 24-hour fast. You can also fast from breakfast to breakfast, or lunch to lunch. The result is the same.

Water, coffee without sugar, and other non-caloric beverages are allowed during the fast, but no solid food. If you are doing this to lose weight, then it is imperative that you eat normal during the eating periods. As in, eat the same amount of food as if you had not been fasting at all. The problem with this method is that a full 24-hour fast can be challenging for many people.

However, you do not need to go all-in right away, starting with 14-16 hours and then moving upwards from there is fine. I do this three times per week. I find the first part of the fast very easy, but in the last few hours, I do become famished, sometimes I would eat dinner early.

The Warrior Diet:

Fitness expert Ori Hofmekler popularized the Warrior Diet. This fasting is a powerful style of Intermittent Fasting and challenging to do. However, it has the highest fat burning benefits. The eating window is 4 hours long, and the fasting window is 20 hours long. You will need to consume all your calories for the day within the 4 hours. If you thought the fast was difficult, consuming all the daily calories within such a short window can be just as difficult. Nevertheless, if you master it, your fat will melt off faster than you ever thought possible.

Even with a fasting plan, you should strive to eat clean and eliminate as much of the poor food choices as you can and replace them with healthier options. Most people nowadays treat food as therapy instead of fuel. They eat even if they are not hungry. That is precisely why obesity is an epidemic. Intermittent Fasting will bring this unhealthy attitude to an abrupt halt. You should eat to live instead of live to eat. Once you achieve this goal, your fat will melt off, and you will reach the body of your dreams.

These three methods are the most popular methods of Intermittent Fasting out there. There are other variations, which involve fasting on alternate days, etc. However, if you are trying to lose weight, the three mentioned above are the best. Pick one that you can manage. That is the most crucial point. Do not pick the hardest one so that you can see quick results. You will probably end up frustrated and quit. So, choose a style that you can handle reasonably well, and stick to it. In 2 to 3 weeks, your body will adapt to the Intermittent Fasting, and within a month, you will be amazed at how much fat you have lost. You have to try Intermittent Fasting to believe it. It is that good.

Five Reasons why Intermittent Fasting increase Weight Loss

Over the past couple of years, Intermittent Fasting has seen its popularity skyrocket as millions of people all over the world have adopted it to lose weight and reclaim their health. It has been proven beyond any doubt to be highly effective for weight loss, and it has several other health benefits too. We will look at five reasons why Intermittent Fasting accelerates fat loss and why it should be something that you should seriously consider adopting if you wish to shed the excess pounds fast.

1. Lowers Inflammation

Inflammation is the leading cause of heart disease and many other health issues. The biggest culprit is sugar, and it creeps into many different foods without you even realizing it. In fact, more people now than ever before have diabetes or are in the prediabetic stage. Intermittent Fasting can reduce inflammation significantly. Since you are only eating during a short eating window, you will not always be feeding your body with detrimental foods throughout the day. As a result, the inflammation in your body will subside. This is very important because when your body is inflamed, it will not burn fat effectively. The cells in your body will not be communicating well with each other due to the inflammation. Intermittent Fasting will set things right, and you will not have an inflamed body to sabotage your fat loss.

2. Promotes Ketosis and Fat Loss

Intermittent Fasting promotes ketosis in the body. Most people have no idea what ketosis is. In simple words, it is the body tapping into the fat stores for fuel. The biggest struggle most people face when losing weight is due to something that occurs that they are not even aware is going on. Your body typically burns glucose for fuel. It gets its glucose from the carbs that you consume. Since people eat from the time they wake to the time they sleep, the body continually has a supply of glucose to burn for fuel. Even if you exercise and watch your diet, it still uses the glucose in your body first. When you are doing Intermittent Fasting, the 16-hour fasting window will ensure that all glucose and glycogen stores are used up in a few hours. Now, your body has no glucose for the remaining hours until you eat next. Therefore, it has no choice but to burn its fat stores for fuel. Now your body is effectively burning fat, and this is why Intermittent Fasting is so powerful. It gets the body to burn the stubborn fat.

3. Stabilizes Blood Sugar Levels

As mentioned earlier, every time you eat, your body will release insulin. This encourages fat storage and prevents your body from burning fat. Intermittent Fasting will ensure that your blood sugar levels are stable and your body can effectively torch the fat without being set back by insulin spikes.

4. Reduce Appetite

Intermittent Fasting will reduce your appetite. When you are fasting for 16 hours a day, your body will adapt and require less food. Maintaining a caloric deficit will become easier, and you will lose the excess weight faster.

5. Increased Energy

Intermittent Fasting has been shown to increase energy levels. That is good news. It means you will be able to perform better during your workouts and burn more calories, which translates to higher overall fat loss. By now, you should be convinced of just how potent Intermittent Fasting is. Make it a part of your lifestyle, and you will never look back.

"BUT GOD, BEING RICH IN MERCY, BECAUSE OF THE GREAT LOVE WITH WHICH HE LOVED US, EVEN WHEN WE WERE DEAD IN OUR TRESPASSES, MADE US ALIVE TOGETHER WITH CHRIST— BY GRACE, YOU HAVE BEEN SAVED."EPHESIANS 2:4-5

FIVE WEIGHT LOSS MYTHS

When it comes to losing weight, there are a lot of misconceptions and just plain half-baked advice out there. Not only can believing them derail your diet efforts, but it can also mess with your health. Have a look at the Weight loss myths below and draw your conclusions.

Myth 1: Crunch and Abdominal Workout Reduce Belly Fat

That statement is false and can hurt your weight loss goals. Exercising your abdominals will help to tone and firm the abdominal region, but it will not reduce fat deposits that are responsible for a potbelly. Fat is reduced uniformly throughout the body there is no such thing as spot reduction. For example, are you eating good calories, or are your calories mainly coming from junk food? You will want to avoid empty calories at all costs; they will only slow down your efforts.

Myth 2: Skipping Breakfast Slows Down Your Metabolism.

Eating breakfast is not essential in a weight-loss plan; Intermittent Fasting is a great way to lose weight. Our body needs time to do what it supposed to do to keep us healthy. We do not need to keep eating, especially if not hungry. At its very core, fasting allows the body to burn off excess body fat. It is important to realize that this is normal and humans have evolved to fast without detrimental health consequences. Body fat is merely food energy that has been stored away. If you do not eat, your body will naturally "eat" its fat for energy.

Myth 3: If it is Fat-Free, I Can Have As Much As I Want.

Unfortunately fat-free doesn't mean calorie free. The word fat-free is misleading because if you overeat on anything, even fat-free foods and you do not burn off those calories, your body will store the excess as fat.

Myth 4: Carbohydrates Make You Gain Weight.

Carbohydrates are an excellent source of energy and necessary for a balanced diet. Choose complex carbohydrates such as fruits, vegetables, and nuts, which are good sources of nutrients (including fiber and B vitamins). Carbohydrates vary widely regarding their nutrient density, so everything from a green bean, which is an excellent source of fiber, protein [and other vitamins and minerals] is considered a carbohydrate," says Pegah Jalali, MS, RD, and CDN. Refined Carbohydrate is the culprit; these carbohydrates are very bad for consumption.

Myth 5: Fat Makes You Fat

First of all, fat is an essential nutrient. An "essential nutrient" is something necessary to life, and even the USDA admits that some amount of saturated fat is necessary to life. Saturated fat helps to form cell membranes all over your body, it's essential for good immune function, it's a fundamental building block for hormones, and it provides energy, they're necessary to life just like magnesium or Vitamin C!)

Cutting out sugar and refined carbs, eating mostly vegetables with some fruit, and then consuming fat (in the form of olive oil, avocados, nuts and seeds, coconut butter, and grass-fed or sustainably and organically raised animal foods) is "the fastest and most effective way to create sustained weight loss says Mark Hyman, MD, director of the Cleveland Clinic Center . If you are consuming saturated fat from these foods, you are not getting "empty calories" by any means: On top of the saturated fat itself, they deliver all kinds of vitamins and minerals – often more than many "low-fat" foods.

In the next chapter, I will be talking about exercise; you may be wondering why I have to talk about exercise since the topic of the book is "How I lost 50 pounds without Exercise." I am not trying to confuse you; exercise is still not needed to lose weight. If I omit activity from this book, it would seem as if I do not think it is essential for our wellbeing. I can't stress this enough; I did not do any form of activity at all while on my weight loss journey.

SHOW ME YOUR WAYS, O LORD. TEACH ME YOUR PATHS. PSALM 25:4

GOD IS OUR REFUGE AND STRENGTH, AN EVER-PRESENT HELP IN TROUBLE. PSALM 46:1

I TRUST IN YOU, O LORD. YOU ARE MY GOD. MY TIMES ARE IN YOUR HAND. PSALM 31: 14-15

BUT SEEK YE FIRST THE KINGDOM OF GOD, AND HIS RIGHTEOUSNESS AND ALL THESE THINGS SHALL BE ADDED UNTO YOU. MATTHEW 6:33

"YET IN ALL THESE THINGS WE ARE MORE THAN CONQUERORS THROUGH HIM WHO LOVED US. FOR I AM PERSUADED THAT NEITHER DEATH NOR LIFE, NOR ANGELS NOR PRINCIPALITIES NOR POWERS, NOR THINGS PRESENT NOR THINGS TO COME, NOR HEIGHT NOR DEPTH, NOR ANY OTHER CREATED THING, SHALL BE ABLE TO SEPARATE US FROM THE LOVE OF GOD WHICH IS IN CHRIST JESUS OUR LORD." **ROMANS 8:37-39**

EXERCISE

You hate to exercise. Okay, so for many, exercise is a bad word. This is common, and it is easy to overcome. Consider changing your mindset. Instead of 'exercise,' call it 'activity.' Find an activity you enjoy. Perhaps you like to bird watch. Going on a weekly bird watching walk is an excellent exercise. Maybe you love to swim or dance. Sign up for a dance class or get a pass to your local pool. Exercise does not mean you have to lift weights and run a marathon. Start by doing something that you love. Get help managing your fitness by exercising with friends. Find an instructor that makes you laugh. Make sure you are having fun and exercise will not feel like exercise.

I never did any exercise during my weight loss journey, but that does not mean I do not think the activity is essential. The point I am trying to make is that we do not need exercise to lose weight. There are many benefits to exercise, everyone benefits from exercise, regardless of age, sex or physical ability. Exercise and physical activity are a great way to feel better and boost your health. Exercise does more than help you burn fat. Exercise stimulates your immune system. It helps increase your metabolism. Remember to check with your doctor before starting a new exercise program, especially if you have not exercised for a long time, have chronic health problems, such as heart disease, diabetes or arthritis, or you have any concerns. Now let us look at some benefits of Exercise.

Controls Weight

Weight loss is the most common benefits to exercise. For most people, losing weight is the reason that they began their exercise program and weight loss can help you avoid many illnesses as well. When you include a healthy diet along with your exercise routine, you are heading toward a more robust body all over. Exercise will burn calories, and when you are taking in fewer calories and burning more, you will lose weight.

Combats Health Conditions and Diseases

The first benefits to exercise that you will discover are the wonderful effect that it will have on your heart and lungs. Exercise will bring more oxygen to every cell in your body and improve the condition of your lungs and heart. The heart will be able to work more efficiently and effectively which will improve the circulation in your whole body. When you increase the strength of your heart and lungs, you will avoid chronic illnesses like stroke, heart attack and breathing problems like asthma.

Improves Mood

One of the benefits to exercise that many people do not realize is the improvement that it causes to your mood. Even people who hate to exercise will find that they are in an excellent mood for the rest of the day when they are finished. When you include exercise in your daily schedule, you will be in an excellent mood all of the time. Not to mention the significant boost to your confidence you will feel when you begin to lose weight.

Boosts Energy

Winded by grocery shopping or household chores? Regular physical activity can improve your muscle strength and boost your endurance. Exercise delivers oxygen and nutrients to your tissues and helps your cardiovascular system work more efficiently. Also, when your heart and lung health improve, you have more energy to tackle daily chores.

Promotes Better Sleep

Regular exercise in your daily schedule can also help you to sleep better. The body will become tired from the exercise, and it will allow you to sleep better when it is time to lie down for the evening. You should make sure that you do not do your exercise right before bed, though, or you will likely keep yourself awake. Plan to do your exercise about three hours at least before bedtime.

So many benefits to exercise will significantly improve your life. You will feel better and look great after just a few weeks of regular exercise. It is one of the greatest natural gifts that you can give to yourself. If you are feeling sluggish, tired and unhappy with your appearance, exercise is the best thing that you can do for your health.

LOVE IS PATIENT, LOVE IS KIND. IT DOES NOT ENVY; IT DOES NOT BOAST, IT IS NOT PROUD. IT DOES NOT DISHONOR OTHERS; IT IS NOT SELF-SEEKING, IT IS NOT EASILY ANGERED, IT KEEPS NO RECORD OF WRONGS. LOVE DOES NOT DELIGHT IN EVIL BUT REJOICES WITH THE TRUTH. IT ALWAYS PROTECTS, ALWAYS TRUSTS, ALWAYS HOPES, ALWAYS PERSEVERES. LOVE NEVER FAILS. BUT WHERE THERE ARE PROPHECIES, THEY WILL CEASE; WHERE THERE ARE TONGUES, THEY WILL BE STILLED; WHERE THERE IS KNOWLEDGE, IT WILL PASS AWAY.

1 CORINTHIANS 13:4-8

RECIPES

As awareness of how wheat affects the body, and the rise of known cases of the Celiac Disease, more and more people are turning to wheat-free diets. Despite the media coverage and ever-growing list of gluten-free products on the market, some folks are still confused about this topic and how they can take part in this ever-growing trend. This short list of recipes will help you get started with your new wheat-free lifestyle. These recipes are Wheat Free, Gluten Free, and Ketogenic (Low Carbohydrates). Please enjoy! These recipes can be eaten anytime during the day. I do not have any particular time to eat. For breakfast, I eat any food, the same for lunch and dinner. If I feel like eating chicken for breakfast, then chicken I will eat, if I feel like having scrambled eggs and bacon for dinner, then that is what I will eat. I always say that my belly does not know the difference, whether it is morning, noon or night.

Ready to live a wheat free life? It is essential to think of food as something that is enjoyable, mainly when you are eliminating something as prevalent as gluten. Some days you might feel like there is nothing you can eat. Make eating a luxurious and delightful endeavor. Add fresh herbs to your meals. Eat foods you have not tasted before and enjoy produce that is bright and colorful. Do not hesitate to try new foods and explore. Moreover, remember to treat yourself to foods that you might miss. For example, make some wheat free cookies, which will help to satisfy that craving.

WHEAT FREE ALMOND FLOUR RAISIN OATMEAL & WALNUT COOKIES

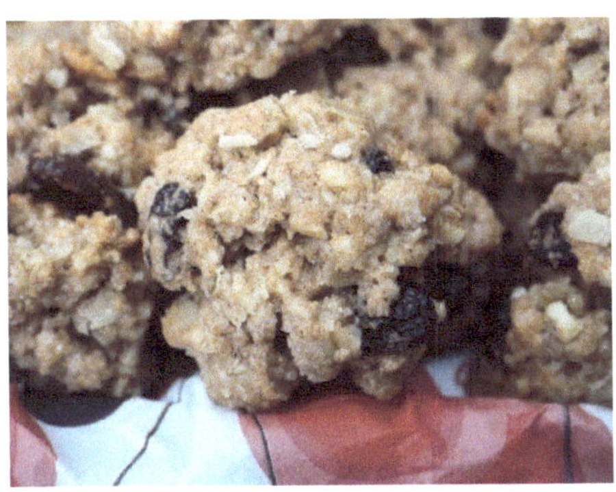

INGREDIENTS

- 3 cups Almond flour
- ½ cup butter (1 stick) softened
- ¼ cup coconut oil
- ½ cup coconut sugar
- 2 large eggs
- ½ tsp baking soda
- 1 ¼ cup raisins
- ½ tsp salt
- 2 tsp vanilla
- 2/3 cup walnuts or oatmeal

DIRECTIONS

1. Preheat oven to 350 degrees, line baking sheet with parchment paper
2. In a bowl cream butter, coconut oil, and Coconut sugar. Add the vanilla and eggs,
3. Mixing until incorporated.
4. Mix baking soda and salt, add the almond flour, 1 cup at a time, beating well of each addition.
5. Fold in the raisins and nuts with a wooden spoon. Form the dough into tablespoon round
6. And place on baking sheet about 3 inches apart. Bake for 13 mins or until golden brown.

7. The dough can be refrigerated for 30 mins before baking.
    Makes about 2 dozen cookies

WHEAT-FREE CREAM CHEESE PANCAKES

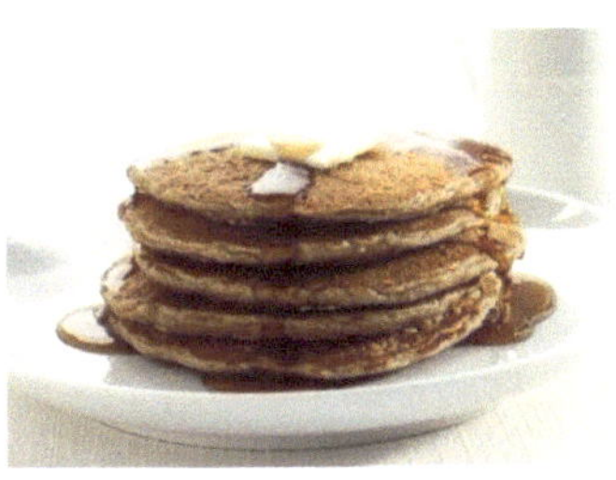

INGREDIENTS

- 2 oz cream cheese
- 2 eggs
- 1 tsp granulated sugar substitute (optional)
- 1/2 tsp cinnamon

DIRECTIONS

1. Put all ingredients in a blender. Blend until smooth.
2. Let rest for 2 minutes so the bubbles can settle.
3. Pour 1/4 of the batter into a hot pan greased with butter.
4. Cook for 2 minutes until golden, flip and cook 1 minute on the other side.
5. Repeat with the rest of the batter.
6. Serve with sugar-free syrup (or Butter) and fresh berries.

WHEAT-FREE CHOCOLATE CHIPS COOKIES

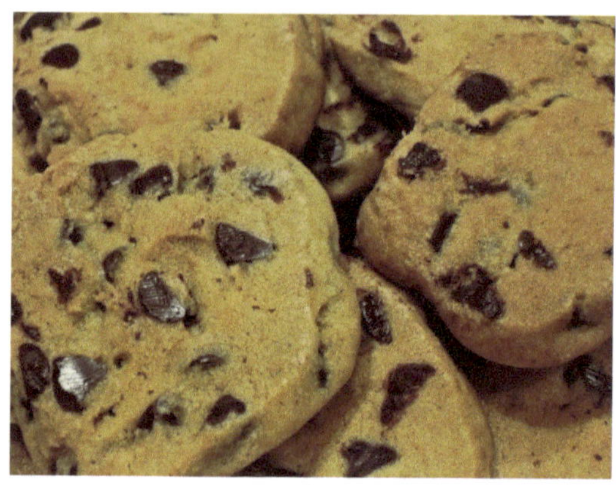

INGREDIENTS
- 1 cup almond flour
- ¼ cup coconut flour
- 1 tsp. baking soda
- 6 tablespoons coconut oil or unsalted butter
- ¾ cup coconut sugar or use sugar substitute (Swerve)
- 1 ½ teaspoons vanilla
- 1 large egg
- 1 ¼ cups sugar-free chocolate chips

DIRECTIONS
1. Preheat oven to 350 degrees, in a medium mixing bowl
2. Stir the dry ingredients and put aside.
3. In a large mixing bowl, beat together fats, and sugar at medium speed until well combined.
4. Add vanilla and beat on medium speed.
5. Beat in egg on low speed and mix until well corporated.
6. Stir in the flour mixture until well combined, and then stir in one cup of chocolate chips.
7. Roll the dough into balls and place on cookie sheet, then put the remaining chips on the top, and the sides flatten with hand.
8. Bake for 11-14 minutes.

WHEAT-FREE COCONUT AND WALNUT BREAD

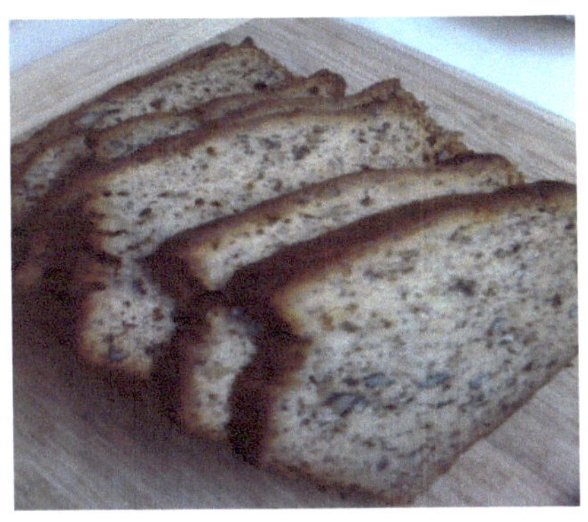

INGREDIENTS

- 2 cups blanched almond flour
- 1/4 cup coconut flour
- 1/4 cup coconut sugar
- 1 tsp baking powder
- 1 tsp baking soda
- 1 tsp cinnamon
- 1/2 tsp salt
- 1/2 cup unsweetened coconut flakes
- 1/3 cup coconut oil melted
- 3 eggs
- 1/2 cup raisin
- 1/2 cup chopped walnuts
- 1 tsp psyllium husk (optional)

DIRECTIONS

1. Preheat your oven to 350 degrees. Generously grease a bread pan and set aside.
2. In a mixing bowl, mix flours, coconut sugar, baking powder & soda, cinnamon, salt and coconut flakes. Set aside.
3. In another bowl, whisk together eggs and coconut oil,
4. Add wet ingredients to dry. Continue to mix and fold until the pockets of dry ingredients are incorporated.

5. Finally, fold in raisins and walnuts, the batter will be thick, pour into the loaf pan. Smooth out the top with a spatula.
6. Bake for 40-45 minutes (depending on oven). Remove from the oven and let sit for at least 15 minutes before removing from the pan.

OVEN JERK CHICKEN (KETOGENIC)

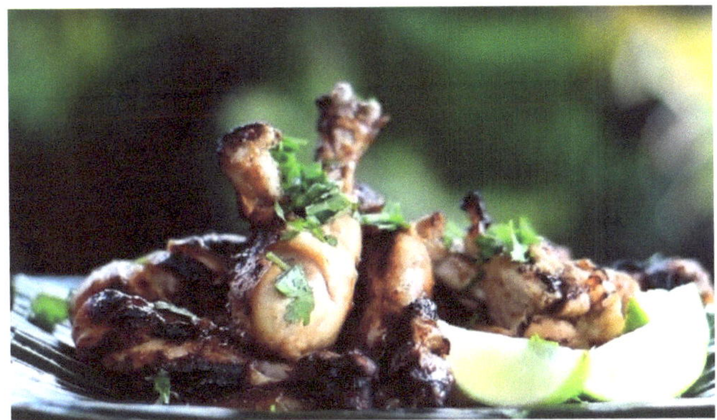

INGREDIENTS FOR JERK CHICKEN

- 2 lbs chicken cut up
- 2 teaspoons salt and pepper or chicken spice
- 1 or more Scotch Bonnet Pepper or any hot pepper
- 5 garlic cloves chopped
- ½ tablespoon allspice coarsely ground
- ½ teaspoon coarsely ground white pepper
- 1 medium onion coarsely chopped
- 4 medium scallions chopped
- 1 sprig of fresh thyme
- 1 tablespoon fresh ginger chopped
- 1 tablespoon Soy Sauce
- 1 tablespoon coconut oil

DIRECTIONS FOR CHICKEN

1. Make the jerk rub by combining all the seasoning.
2. Toss the chicken pieces with the spice mixture
3. Cover, and marinate in the refrigerator 2 to 4 hours. Marinate overnight is better.

1. Preheat oven to 350 degrees F (175 degrees C).
2. Pour the coconut oil into a 9x13 inch baking dish.
3. Place the chicken pieces skin-side up into the baking dish.
4. Bake in the preheated oven for 1 hour 20 minutes, until no longer pink near the bone.
5. Turn the oven on to broil, and cook until the skin crisps, 2 to 5 minutes

You can eat any form of steam vegetables or salad with this recipe.

JAMAICAN ESCOVITCH FISH (KETOGENIC)

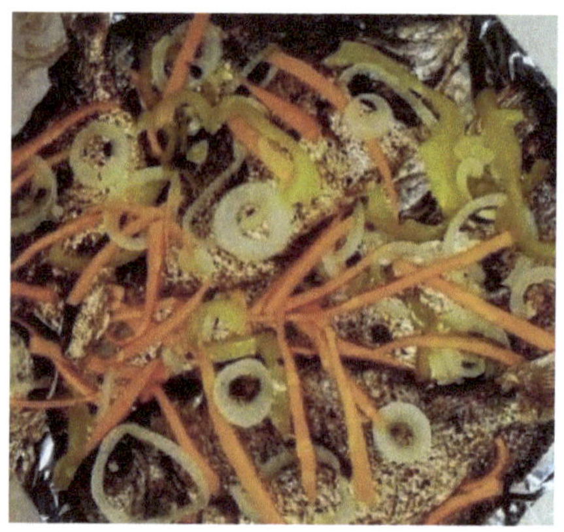

INGREDIENTS

- 2 pounds whole red snapper about 2-3 fish or any white fish – cleaned and scaled.
- ½ cup coconut oil or more as needed
- 1 teaspoon minced garlic about 2 garlic cloves
- ½ teaspoon ginger
- 2 sprigs thyme
- 1 yellow medium onion thinly sliced

- 1 medium carrot cut into long strips
- ½ teaspoon Jamaican allspice
- 1 Scotch bonnet pepper pierced or replace with ½ teaspoon cayenne pepper
- ¾ cup malt vinegar sub red wine vinegar
- Freshly ground white pepper

DIRECTIONS

1. Rinse fish; rub with lemon or lime.
2. Season with salt and pepper or use your favorite seasoning.
3. In a large skillet heat oil over medium heat until hot
4. Add the fish and cook each side- for about 5-7 minutes until cooked through and crispy on both sides.
5. Remove fish and set aside. Drain oil and leave about 2-3 tablespoons of oil
6. Add garlic and ginger, stir-fry for about a minute making sure the garlic does not burn
7. Add onion, thyme, scotch bonnet, and all spice-continue stirring for about 2-3 minutes.
8. Add vinegar, mix an adjust salt and pepper according to preference. Let it simmer for about 2 more minutes.
9. Discard thyme sprig and serve over the fish. You may make the sauce about 2 days in advance.

You can eat any form of steam vegetables or salad with this recipe.

KETOGENIC CREAMY CABBAGE SALAD

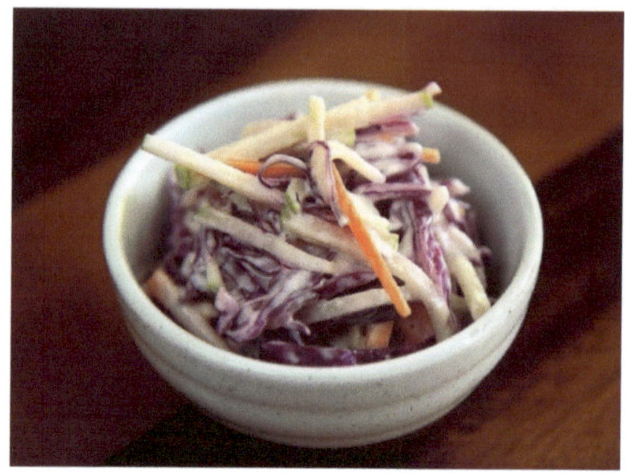

INGREDIENTS

- 1/2 head purple or green cabbage, thinly sliced
- 2 large carrots thinly sliced
- 1/4 cup mayonnaise
- 1/2 cup yogurt, full fat
- 1/2 teaspoon sea salt
- 1 teaspoon ginger, ground

DIRECTIONS

1. In a large salad bowl, mix cabbage and carrot slices, mayonnaise, yogurt, sea salt, ginger.
2. Toss well to distribute the salt and ginger evenly
3. Cover & allow chilling overnight in the refrigerator.

WHEAT-FREE FRIED CHICKEN

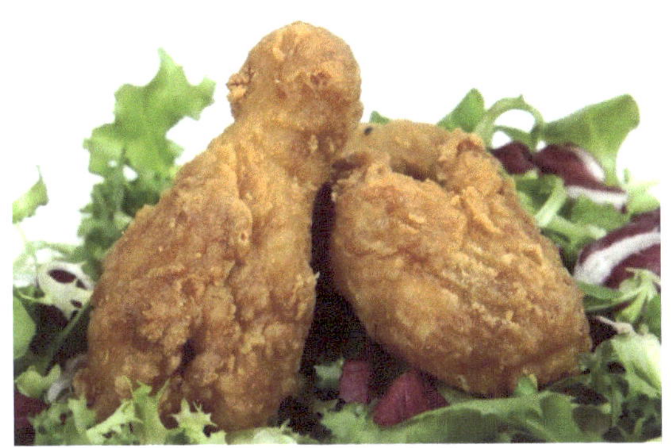

INGREDIENTS

- 1 whole chicken cut into 10 pieces
- 1 1/2 – 2 teaspoons salt adjust to preference
- 3-4 garlic crushed
- 2-3 teaspoons all-purpose seasoning
- 3 cups Almond Flour, Parmesan Cheese or (gluten-free flour)
- 1 tablespoon paprika
- 1 teaspoon salt adjust to taste
- 2 tablespoon garlic powder
- 2 tablespoon onion powder
- 1 teaspoon cayenne pepper
- 1 teaspoon white pepper
- 2 large eggs beaten

DIRECTIONS

1. Place chicken in a large bowl or Large Ziploc. Then seasoned with salt followed by all the crushed garlic, hot sauce, and all-purpose seasoning

2. If desired, transfer the chicken to a gallon-sized zipper-lock freezer bag and refrigerate for at least 4 hours and up to overnight.
3. In a large bowl, whisk together the flour, salt, paprika, garlic powder, onion powder, cayenne pepper, herbs and white pepper.
4. In a large bowl beat eggs, add a little salt. Dip chicken in egg mixture.
5. Dredge chicken in flour mixture, shaking any excess flour. You may use a Ziploc bag for this process, too.
6. Set aside for about 10-15 minutes while preparing oil. Doing so will help the coating to stay on better
7. .

FRYING THE CHICKEN

1. Heat oil in a deep fryer or cast iron skillet to 375 degrees F (190 degrees C). The temperature will drop once you add chicken.
2. Using a tong and carefully and slowly place the chicken in the hot oil. Work in batches. Do not overcrowd the skillet.
3. Fry the chicken until golden brown, turning once every 8 to 15 minutes - depending on the size of the pieces. Chicken is done when it is no longer pink inside, and its juices run clear. You may do a test by piercing the chicken with a fork.
4. Drain the chicken on paper towels and then transfer them to a wire rack.

You can eat any form of steam vegetables or salad with this recipe.

JAMAICAN OXTAIL STEW (KETOGENIC)

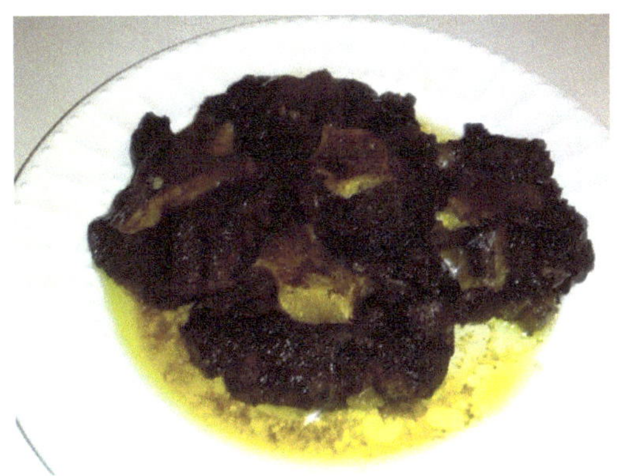

INGREDIENTS

- 2 -3 tablespoon coconut or olive oil
- 2 pounds oxtail cut up medium pieces
- 1 onion chopped
- 2 teaspoon minced garlic
- teaspoon fresh chopped thyme
- 1 Whole Scotch bonnet pepper
- 2 green onions chopped
- 5-6 Whole pimento seeds (allspice),
- 1 Tablespoon gravy master for coloring
- Salt to taste

DIRECTIONS

1. Season oxtail with, salt and pepper. Set aside
2. In a large pot, heat oil over medium heat, until hot, and then add the oxtail sauté stirring, frequently, until oxtail is brown. If desire drain the oil and leave about 2-3 tablespoons
3. Add onions, green onions, garlic, thyme, allspice, gravy master, stir for about a minute. Throw in scotch bonnet pepper, stir for another minute.

4. Then add about 4-6 cups of water, it is best to start with 4 cups, and then add as needed. Bring to a boil and let it simmer until tender (depending on the oxtail size and preference) about 2- 3 hours, occasionally stirring the saucepan.
5. Adjust the thickness of gravy with water or stock; if the sauce is too thin, you can thicken with flaxseed meal.
6. Season with salt according to preference.

You can eat any form of steam vegetables or salad with this recipe.

WHEAT-FREE PIZZA WITH CHEESE CRUST

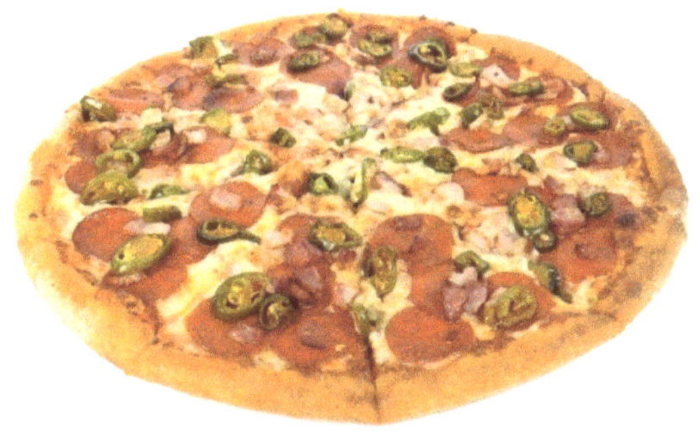

INGREDIENTS
- 1 1/2 cup Mozzarella cheese (shredded)
- 2 tbsp Cream cheese (cut into cubes)
- 2 large Egg (beaten)
- 1/3 cup Almond Flour

DIRECTIONS
1. Preheat the oven to 425 degrees F. Line a baking sheet or pizza pan with parchment paper.
2. Combine the shredded mozzarella and cubed cream cheese in a large bowl. Microwave for 90 seconds, stirring halfway through. Stir again at the end until well incorporated.
3. Stir in the beaten eggs and Almond Flour. Knead with your hands until a dough forms. If the dough becomes hard before thoroughly mixed, you can microwave for 10-15 seconds to soften it.
4. Spread the dough onto the lined baking pan to 1/4" or 1/3" thickness, using your hands or a rolling pin over a piece of parchment (the rolling pin works better if you have one). Use a toothpick or fork to poke lots of holes throughout the crust to prevent bubbling.

5. Bake for 6 minutes. Poke more holes in any places where you see bubbles forming. Bake for 3-7 more minutes, until golden brown.
6. To make keto pizza, top with Cheese, sauce, Chicken, and pepper after cooking the crust and return to the oven for about 10 minutes, until thoroughly heated.
7. You can use any topping you like

WHEAT-FREE BISCUIT

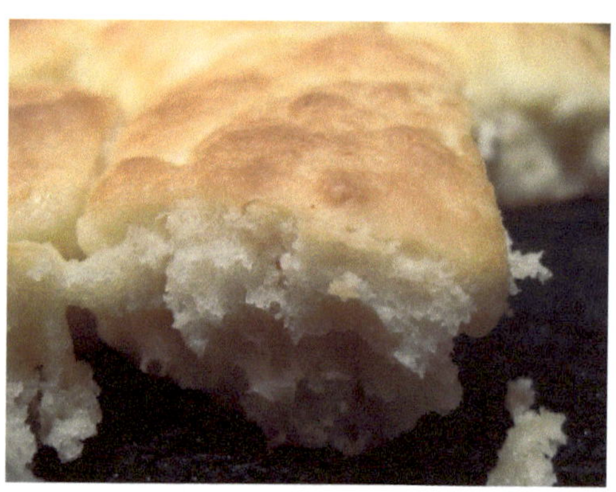

INGREDIENTS
- 2 1/2 cups blanched almond flour, for biscuits
- 1 cup blanched almond flour, for dusting the dough
- 1/2 teaspoon Celtic sea salt
- 1/2 teaspoon baking soda
- 1/4 cup coconut oil
- 2 eggs
- 1 tablespoon honey

DIRECTIONS
1. Combine almond flour, salt and baking soda in a medium bowl
2. Blend coconut oil, eggs, and honey in a large bowl

3. Stir the dry ingredients and the wet ones together until a nice dough forms
4. Between 2 pieces of parchment paper, roll out dough to 3/4 inch thickness
5. If the dough is sticky, dust dough with extra almond flour
6. Using a mason jar with a 2 1/2 inch wide mouth, cut the dough into biscuits
7. Using a spatula, transfer biscuits to a parchment lined a baking sheet
8. Preheat oven to 350 degrees Fahrenheit
9. Bake biscuits until browned on the bottom edges, about 15 minutes
10. Serve fresh, hot biscuits with butter, jelly, gravy, or anything else that sounds good

FREE BONUS

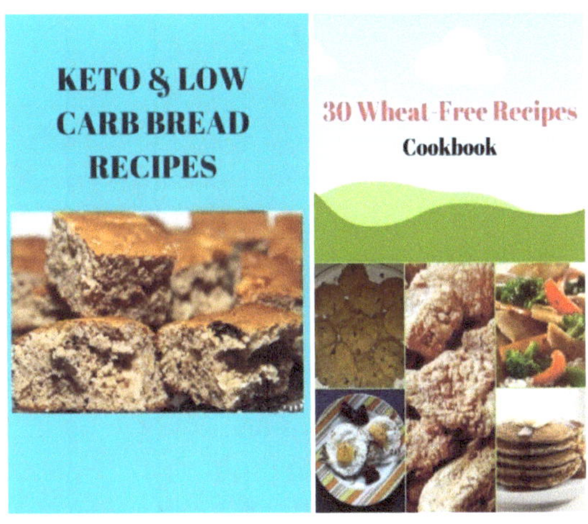

Get it for FREE. Please email me at howilost50pounds@gmail.com to get the link to download now.

CONCLUSION

Many people think that being overweight is just an appearance issue. However, being overweight is a medical concern because it can seriously affect a person's health. The health problems that stem from being overweight go way beyond the ones we usually hear about, like diabetes and heart disease. Here are some other issues with being overweight can cause.

Arthritis. Wear and tear on the joints from carrying extra weight can cause this painful joint problem even at a young age.

Sleep Apnea. This condition (where a person temporarily stops breathing during sleep) is a severe problem for many overweight kids and adults. Not only does it interrupt sleep, but sleep apnea can also leave people feeling tired and affect their ability to concentrate and learn. It also may lead to heart problems.

Asthma. Obesity associated with breathing problems that can make it harder to keep up with friends, play sports, or walk from class to class.

High Blood Pressure. When blood pressure is high, the heart must pump harder, and the arteries must carry blood that is moving under greater pressure. If the problem continues for a long time, the heart and arteries may no longer work as well as they should. High blood pressure, or hypertension, is more common in overweight or obese teens.

These are only a few of the problems being overweight can cause. I am happy that I took steps to lose weight; I am healthier, and I feel better and look great. It took me a while, but it worth all the sacrifices I made. If I can do it, anyone can. I never thought I could lose so much weight. I did not deprive myself, and I was not hungry. Please implement the three methods I mentioned in your life, and you will not regret it. Also, it is critically important that you maintain a positive attitude. Be forgiving of yourself. If you veer off your diet plan, get back on course with your next meal.

Do not spend precious time "beating yourself up" over your failures. Instead, celebrate your successes in a non-fattening way. For instance, when you reach a milestone, say you have lost ten pounds reward yourself with a trip to an art museum or your favorite coffee shop (but skip the sugar). Marking milestones will give you a sense of accomplishment, a feeling that you are triumphing over food.

You will have great success. I wish you all the best of luck, and I would like to hear about your successful weight loss journey someday. You are not alone; I am with you in spirit. God bless you all. You can do all things through Christ who strengthens you.

Many thanks for purchasing and reading my book. I know there are numerous other books out there and that your time and effort is valuable, therefore; I am very grateful that you had taken the time to read my book. If you enjoyed the book, please consider leaving a review on Amazon. I would appreciate it. All the best on your weight loss journey also to a healthier you. God Bless You!

Love
Annett Hill

PEACE I LEAVE WITH YOU; MY PEACE I GIVE TO YOU; NOT AS THE WORLD GIVES DO I GIVE TO YOU. LET NOT YOUR HEART BE TROUBLED, NEITHER LET IT BE AFRAID. JOHN 14:27